The Sirtfood Diet

Lose weight naturally and activate your
SKINNY GENE
with healthy and delicious recipes

Lisa T. Oliver

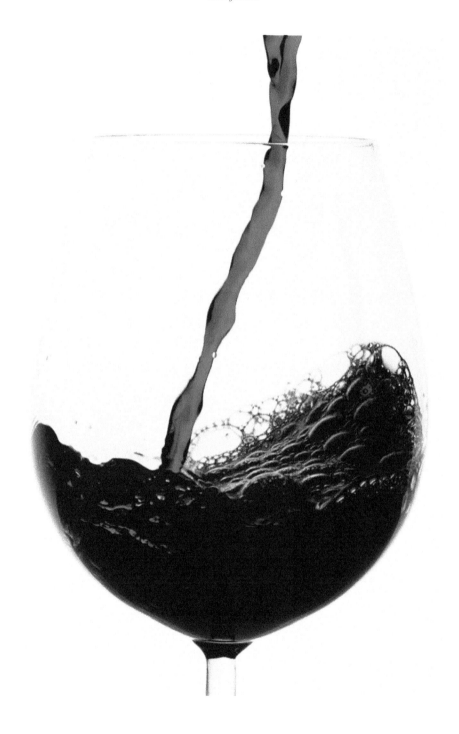

© Copyright 2021 All rights reserved.

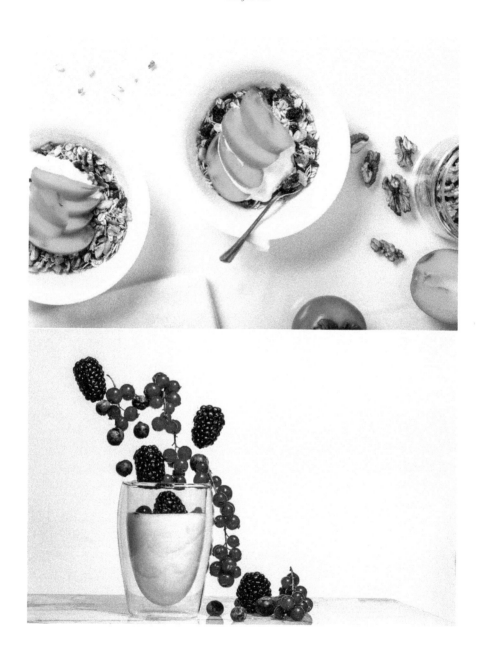

Contents

Introduction

The Sirtfood Diet, launched in 2016, has been a trending topic for a while now, with people following the diet very strictly. The creators of the diet suggest that these foods function by activating proteins in the body, referred to as sirtuins. The idea is that sirtuins protect body cells from dying when subjected to stress and regulate metabolism, inflammation, and aging. Sirtuins also boost the body's metabolism and affect its ability to burn fat, providing a weight loss of about seven pounds in a week while retaining muscle. Nonetheless, experts believe that this is solely about fat loss rather than differences in glycogen storage from the liver and skeletal muscle. This diet was developed by UK-based nutritionists, both with MAs in nutritional medicine, and has since gained popularity among athletes and celebrities. Adele and Pippa Middleton are two celebrities who have followed the Sirtfood Diet, and it yielded great results for them. The Sirtfood Diet, like most diets, promotes sustained and significant weight loss, improved health, and better energy. What is it about this diet? Is it just a fad, or is there more to it? Does science back it up? All these questions and more will be answered as you read on. The word "sirt" comes from sirtuins, a group of Silent Information Regulator (SIR) proteins. They boost metabolism, improve muscle efficiency, reduce inflammation, and start the process of fat loss and cell repair. These sirtuins make us healthier, fit, and also help in fighting diseases. Exercise and restrictions on calorie consumption improve sirtuin production in the body.

The Premise of the Sirtfood Diet The premise of the Sirtfood Diet states that certain foods can mimic the benefits of fasting and caloric restrictions by activating sirtuins, which are proteins in the body. They range from SIRT1 to SIRT7, switch genes on and off, maintain biological pathways, and protect cells from age-related decline. Although intense calorie restriction and fasting are severe, the Sirtfood Diet inventors developed a plan with a focus on eating plenty of sirtfoods. It's a more natural way to stimulate sirtuin genes in the body, also known as skinny genes. In the process, it improves health and boosts weight loss. If you want to start the Sirtfood Diet, planning is required, and access to the ingredients needed to follow the diet correctly. There are many exciting recipes for the diet, with a variety of ingredients. However, it may often be challenging to get certain ingredients during specific seasons and times of the year. Some of these ingredients include kale and strawberries, for example. It may also be stressful to follow social events when traveling or to care for a young child. The Sirtfood Diet covers various food groups; however, dairy foods aren't included in the plan. Sirtfoods are a new diet discovery. They are rich in nutrients and capable of activating skinny genes in the body, with benefits and downsides alike.

CHAPTER 1: THE SCIENCE OF SIRTUINS

The Sirtfood diet is very famous due to its scientific benefits and amazing transformations within the body's metabolic capacities. Thousands of people have unlocked incredible and aesthetic physiques by following the Sirtfood diet. These results are not coming from word of mouth or myths attached to basic philosophies of dieting; in fact, the Sirtfood diet has a robust yet growing scientific background. The discovery of the Sirtfood diet was not an accident, but researchers found the necessary components, the polyphenols, in labs and conducted many types of research to conform to the scientific benefits of the Sirtfood diet. The primary lean gene, also known as a sirtuin, on which this dieting style got its name was first found in 1984 and not in humans but in yeasts. Polyphenol is a well-known chemical compound present in the body and acts on an essential lean gene to activate and perform fat-burning blitz inside the human body. To be very specific, Sirtfoods are those which contain high levels of a chemical compound called polyphenol. This compound is not uniformly distributed in Sirtfoods, but every Sirtfood contains specific amounts of polyphenols. The answer is straightforward yet very informative. Polyphenols are the compounds that are present naturally in Sirtfood, and many types of research conducted have confirmed that these foods have the highest impacts when losing extra pounds of fats from the body.

Polyphenols are essential precursors in the fat burning cycle of the body called lipolysis. Free fatty acids in our blood are subjected to digestion and then excretion from the body through an enzyme called lipase. Foods rich in Polyphenols cause much increase in levels of lipase enzyme and thus more fat burning blitz in the body. Polyphenols act on lipase and other fat-burning mediators by activating a particular type of gene in the body called sirtuin. This gene is the most crucial part of the Sirtfood diet because, through this gene activation, polyphenol-rich foods called the Sirtfoods act on extra stored fat in our body and engine a fat-burning cycle in our body to get rid of it. Sirtuin gene is a human gene and present in every human. It is also present in some other animals as well but in modified forms. Interestingly, the very first encounter with the sirtuin gene was in 2002 when a group of researchers found its over-activation associated with particular types of foods given to some animals. Then many studies were conducted on mice to check the efficacy of these foods and the activation of the sirtuin gene in the human body. These trials confirmed that the sirtuin gene is associated with fat loss, and Sirtfoods, which contain the maximum amount of polyphenol, are very important when undergoing a fat loss diet.

It is also fascinating to know that Sirtfoods are not very rare types of food. These foods contain a significant portion of both eastern and western diets as well as in Mediterranean diets. The Sirtfood diet consists of the top twenty foods in the world, which are considered as the basic Sirtfoods. These twenty foods contain the highest amounts of sirtuin-activating polyphenols. The levels of polyphenol are not uniformly distributed in all these foods, and some of them contain higher amounts. Moreover, different types of polyphenols are present in these Sirtfoods, which are associated with special effects on the sirtuin gene. The most important aspect of the Sirtfood diet is that it uses a variety of foods. These twenty Sirtfoods make an essential part of the Sirtfood diet so that the maximum amount of all types of polyphenols is consumed to maximize the fat burning in our body.

CHAPTER 2: The Science Behind the Fat-Burning Benefits of the Sirtfood Diet

The most significant benefit of the Sirtfood diet is its incredible impact on losing fats from the body. Fats are made up of fatty acids that combine to make adipocytes. These adipocytes are clusters of fatty acids, and unlike free fatty acids, adipocytes are not mostly present in the blood. They get accumulated under the skin, in muscles, and on different organs. These adipocytes combine to make adipose tissues, which are full fledge foam-shaped cluster of visible yellowish white-color fat in our body. Adipocytes are the healthiest fat cells to burn, and they must have been broken down into adipocytes and finally in free fatty acids (in reverse order of formation) to get burned from the fat-burning enzymes called the lipase enzyme. These steps are not easy as they seem, and burning extra pounds of fats can be a hard nut to crack. The most challenging step in this cycle is to break adipose tissues in adipocytes. The Sirtfoods contain high levels of polyphenols.

CHAPTER 3: The Sirtfood Diet and Energy Cycle of the Body

The fuel of the body is glucose, which is the most readily available nutrient in the body for energy. The glucose is broken down into energy packets called ATPs, which are produced from the power of cells called mitochondria. These energy packets are utilized to fuel the body while performing actions. High-intensity work such as exercise requires a much more significant amount of energy as compared to typing on a keyboard. The higher the intensity of work, the larger will be the needed number of ATPs. The most significant source of glucose in the body is carbohydrates, which are sugars in simpler forms. A diet rich in low glycemic carbohydrates is essential while performing high-intensity tasks. These carbohydrates are broken down into the purest form of sugar called glucose. This glucose undergoes a series of reactions called glycolysis. In this cycle, the end product is the ATPs that are stored or utilized in response to stress produced in the body. These ATPs are also crucial for fighting against the infections because the higher the level of energy in the body, the greater will be the immune response of the body. All the processes are directly proportional.

The Sirtfood diet is affluent in proteins, good fats, and low glycemic carbohydrates. All these macronutrients are essential for fulfilling the body's essential needs of energy and refueling.

CHAPTER 4: The Sirtfood Diet and Poke Hole Theory

This is by far the most valuable information about the Sirtfood diet. Very brief literature is available about the poke hole theory and its relationship with the Sirtfood diet. When a person undergoes a diet, which comprises of a calorie deficit scenario, our body takes it as a challenge and signals our mitochondria—the powerhouse of the cell to produce ATP, which are the energy packets to supply the body with instant energy. This calorie deficit scenario pokes holes in mitochondria, and thus, specific genes are activated in a cyclic manner to produce a considerable amount of energy in response to these holes in mitochondria. You can say that mitochondria get excited in response to these poked holes. A significant benefit of this cycling production of energy is the utilization of stored fats as a source of energy. When the body is not getting enough from outside sources, it becomes evident that the body must utilize its energy stores either from fat, muscles, or available glucose.

As the energy consumption is higher and calorie intake is higher when someone starts a calorie deficit diet such as the Sirtfood diet, the body acts on cyclic use of its stored fat to mobilize it in blood, and high metabolic rates due to exercise cause consumption and immediate burning of these free fatty acids in the blood. If someone consumes fat mobilizing precursors from the diet, this fat-burning mechanism can speed up too many folds.

CHAPTER 5:

Breakfast

1.   Blueberry Frozen Yogurt

Preparation Time: 15 minutes

Cooking Time: 0 minutes

Servings: 4

Ingredients:

450g (1lb) plain yogurt

175g (6oz) blueberries

Juice of 1 orange

One tablespoon honey

Directions:

Place the blueberries and orange juice into a food processor or blender and blitz until smooth.

Press the mixture through a sieve into a large bowl to remove seeds. Stir in the honey and yogurt. Transfer the mixture to an ice-cream maker and follow the manufacturer's instructions.

Alternatively, pour the mixture into a container and place in the fridge for 1 hour. Use a fork to whisk it and break up ice crystals and freeze for 2 hours.

Nutrition:

Energy (calories): 483 kcal

Protein: 47.06 g Fat: 2.33g

Carbohydrates: 72.11 g

2. Hearty Almond Crackers

Preparation time: 10 minutes

Cooking Time: 20 minutes

Servings: 40

Ingredients:

1 cup almond flour

¼ teaspoon baking soda

1/8 teaspoon black pepper

Three tablespoons sesame seeds

One egg, beaten

Salt and pepper to taste

Directions:

Preheat your oven to 350 degrees F.

Line two baking sheets with parchment paper and keep them on the side.

Mix the dry ingredients in a large bowl and add egg, mix well and form the dough.

Divide dough into two balls.

Roll out the dough between two pieces of parchment paper.

Cut into crackers and transfer them to the prepared baking sheet.

Bake for 15-20 minutes.

Repeat until all the dough is used up.

Leave crackers to cool and serve.

Enjoy!

Nutrition:

Total Carbs: 8g Fiber: 2g

Protein: 9g

Fat: 28g

3.   Strawberry And Cherry Smoothie

Preparation Time: 3 minutes

Cooking Time: 0 minute

Servings: 1

Ingredients:

100g (3½ oz.) strawberries

75g (3oz) frozen pitted cherries

One tablespoon plain full-fat yogurt

175mls (6fl oz.) unsweetened soya milk

Directions:

Place all the ingredients into a blender and process until smooth. Serve and enjoy.

Nutrition:

Energy (calories): 108 kcal

Protein: 2.34 g Fat: 0.63 g

Carbohydrates: 25.53 g

4.   Eggs With Kale

Preparation Time: 2 minutes

Cooking Time: 1 minute

Servings: 1

Ingredients:

Two large eggs

Salt

Ground black pepper

1 tsp. olive oil or avocado oil

1 cup kale

Directions:

Heat 1 tsp. Olive oil in the skillet over (medium/high) heat. Add kale and cook, tossing, until wilted (approx. 1 minute). Remove kale, add eggs, and fry until done. Serve with kale.

Nutrition:

Calories: 136.4 g

Total Fat: 8.4 g

Total Carbs: 7.9 g

Sugars: 1.6 g Protein: 8.7 g

5.　　Moroccan Spiced Eggs

Preparation time: 1 hour

Cooking time: 50 minutes

Servings: 2

Ingredients:

1 tsp. olive oil

One shallot, stripped and finely hacked

One red (chime) pepper, deseeded and finely hacked

One garlic clove, stripped and finely hacked

One courgette (zucchini), stripped and finely hacked

½ tsp. gentle stew powder

½ tsp. salt

One × 400g (14oz) can hacked tomatoes

1 x 400g (14oz) may need chickpeas in water

a little bunch of level leaf parsley (10g (1/3oz)), cleaved

Four medium eggs at room temperature

Directions:

Heat the oil in a pan; include the shallot and red (ringer) pepper and fry delicately for 5 minutes. At that point, have the garlic and courgette (zucchini) and cook for one more moment or two. Include the tomato puree (glue), flavors, and salt and mix through.

Add the cleaved tomatoes and chickpeas (dousing alcohol and all) and increment the warmth to medium.

Stew the sauce for 30 minutes.

Ensure it is delicately rising all through and permit it to lessen in volume by around 33%.

Remove from the warmth and mix in the cleaved parsley.

Preheat the grill to 200C/180C fan/350F.

When you are prepared to cook the eggs, bring the tomato sauce up to a delicate stew and move to a little broiler confirmation dish.

Crack the eggs on the dish and lower them delicately into the stew. Spread with thwart and prepare in the grill for 10-15 minutes. Serve the blend in unique words with the eggs coasting on the top.

Nutrition:

Calories: 116 kcal

Protein: 6.97 g Fat: 5.22 g

Carbohydrates: 13.14 g

6.   Twice Baked Breakfast Potatoes

Preparation time: 10 minutes

Cooking time: 1 hour

Servings: 2

Ingredients:

Two medium reddish brown potatoes, cleaned and pricked with a fork everywhere

Two tablespoons unsalted spread

Three tablespoons overwhelming cream

Four rashers cooked bacon

Four huge eggs

½ cup destroyed cheddar

Daintily cut chives

Salt and pepper to taste

Directions:

Preheat grill to 400°F.

Spot potatoes straightforwardly on the stove rack in the grill's focal point and prepare for 30 to 45 min.

Evacuate and permit potatoes to cool for around 15 minutes.

Cut every potato down the middle longwise and burrow every half out, scooping the potato substance into a blending bowl.

Gather margarine and cream to the potato and pound into a single unit until smooth — season with salt and pepper and mix.

Spread a portion of the potato blend into each emptied potato skin base and sprinkle with one tablespoon cheddar (you may make them remain pounded potato left to snack on).

Add one rasher bacon to every half and top with a raw egg.

Spot potatoes onto a heating sheet and come back to the appliance.

Lower broiler temperature to 375°F and heat potatoes until egg whites are simply set and yolks are as yet runny.

Top every potato with a sprinkle of the rest of the cheddar, season with salt and pepper, and finish with cut chives.

Nutrition:

Calories: 647 kcal

Protein: 30.46 g

Fat: 55.79 g

Carbohydrates: 7.45 g

7.   Sirt Muesli

Preparation time: 30 minutes

Cooking time: 0 minutes

Servings: 2

Ingredients:

Directions:

Blend the entirety of the above fixings (forget about the strawberries and yogurt if not serving straight away).

Nutrition:

Calories: 334 kcal

Protein: 4.39 g

Fat: 22.58 g

Carbohydrates: 34.35 g

8.   Blueberry Muffins

Preparation time: 15 minutes

Cooking time: 20 minutes

Servings: 8

Ingredients

1 cup buckwheat flour

1½ teaspoons baking powder

¼ teaspoon of sea salt

Two eggs

½ cup unsweetened almond milk

2–3 tablespoons maple syrup

Two tablespoons coconut oil, melted

1 cup fresh blueberries

Directions:

Preheat your oven to 350°F and line 8 cups of a muffin tin.

In a bowl, place the buckwheat flour, baking powder, and salt, and mix well.

Place the eggs, almond milk, maple syrup, and coconut oil and beat until well combined in a separate bowl.

Now, place the flour mixture and mix until just combined.

Gently fold in the blueberries.

Transfer the mixture into prepared muffin cups evenly.

Bake for about 25 minutes or until a toothpick inserted in the center comes out clean.

Remove the muffin tin from the oven and place it onto a wire rack to cool for about 10 minutes.

Carefully invert the muffins onto the wire rack to cool completely before serving.

Nutrition:

Calories 136

Fat 5.3 g

Carbs 20.7 g

Protein 3.5 g

9.   Easy Egg-White Muffins

Preparation time: 10 minutes

Cooking time: 15 minutes

Servings: 2

Ingredients

English muffin - I enjoy Ezekiel 7 grain

Egg-whites - 6 tbsp. or two large egg whites

Turkey bacon or bacon sausage

Sharp cheddar cheese or gouda

Organic berry

Optional-lettuce and hot sauce, hummus, flaxseeds

Directions:

Get a microwavable safe container, then spray entirely to stop the egg from adhering, then pour egg whites into the dish.

Lay turkey bacon or bacon sausage paper towel and then cook.

Subsequently, toast your muffin, if preferred.

Then put the egg dish in the microwave for 30 minutes. Afterward, with a spoon or fork, immediately flip the egg within the plate and cook for another 30 minutes.

While the dish remains hot, sprinkle some cheese while preparing sausage.

The secret is to get a paste of some kind between each coating to put up the sandwich together, i.e., a tiny little bit of hummus or even cheese.

Nutrition:

Energy (calories): 1109 kcal

Protein: 47.01 g

Fat: 8.39 g

Carbohydrates: 214.24 g

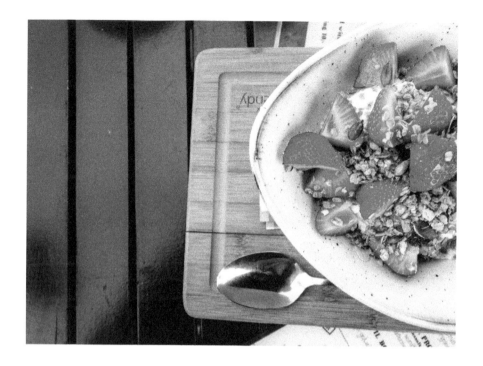

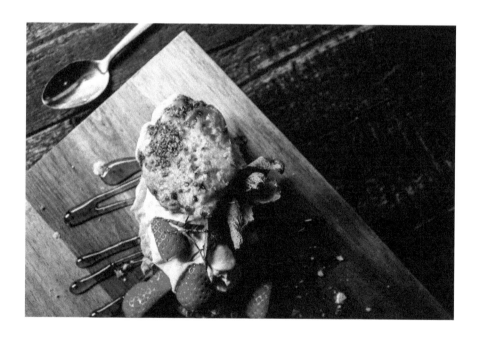

CHAPTER 6:

Lunch

10.   Muesli Sirt

You just add the dry ingredients and put the mixture in an airtight jar if you want to make this in bulk or cook it the night before. The next day all you have to do is add the strawberries and milk, and it's ready to go.

Preparation Time: 20 min.

Cooking Time: 0 minute

Servings: 2

Ingredients:

Buckwheat flakes: 1/4 cup (20 g)

Buckwheat puffs: 2/3 cup (10 g)

3 Tablespoons (15 g) of coconut or dry cocoa flakes

Cup 1/4 (40 g) Medjool seeds, diced and pitted

1/8 cup (15 g) chopped walnuts

11/2 cups (10 g) of cocoa nibs

2/3 cup (100 g) hulled and chopped strawberries

Pure Greek yogurt (or vegan substitute, such as soy or coconut yogurt) 3/8 cup (100 g)

Directions:

Mix all the ingredients (leave off the strawberries and cream, if not instantly served).

Nutrition:

Energy (calories): 1559 kcal

Protein: 100.84 g

Fat: 92.45 g

Carbohydrates: 330.67 g

11. Salmon And Spinach Quiche

Preparation time: 55 minutes

Cooking time: 45 minutes

Servings: 2

Ingredients

600 g (21 oz.) frozen leaf spinach

One clove of garlic

One onion

150 g (5 ¼ oz.) frozen salmon fillets

200 g (7 oz.) smoked salmon

One small bunch of dill

One untreated lemon

50 g (1 ⅝ oz.) butter

200 g (7 oz.) sour cream

Three eggs

Salt, pepper, nutmeg

One pack of puff pastry

Directions

Let the spinach thaw and squeeze well.

Peel the garlic and onion and cut into fine cubes.

Cut the salmon fillet into cubes 1-1.5 cm (0.40-0.60 inch) thick.

Cut the smoked salmon into strips.

Wash the dill, pat dry and chop.

Wash the lemon with hot water, dry, rub the zest finely with a kitchen grater, and squeeze the lemon.

Heat the butter in a pan. Sweat the garlic and onion cubes in it for approx. 2-3 minutes.

Add spinach and sweat briefly.

Add sour cream, lemon juice, and zest, eggs, and dill and mix well.

Season with salt, pepper, and nutmeg.

Preheat the oven to 200°C (390°F).

Grease a spring form pan and roll out the puff pastry in it and pull up on edge. Prick the dough with a fork (so that it doesn't rise too much).

Pour in the spinach and egg mixture and smooth out.

Spread the salmon cubes and smoked salmon strips on top.

The quiche in the oven (grid, middle inset) about 30-40 min. Yellow gold bakes.

NutritionCalories: 903 kcalProtein: 65.28 gFat: 59.79 gCarbohydrates: 30.79 g

12.   Turmeric Chicken & Kale Salad With Honey Lime Dressing

Preparation time: 55 minutes

Cooking time: 20 minutes

Servings: 2

Ingredients

For chicken

One teaspoon ghee or one tablespoon of coconut oil

½ medium brown onion, diced

250-300 g (9 oz.) Ground chicken or cubed chicken thighs

One large clove of garlic, finely diced

One teaspoon turmeric powder

One teaspoon lime zest

½ lime juice

½ tsp. salt + pepper

For salad

Six stems of broccoli or 2 cups of broccoli florets

Two tablespoons of pumpkin seeds

Three large kale leaves stem removed and chopped

½ Avocado, slice

A handful of fresh coriander leaves, chopped

A handful of fresh parsley leaves chopped

For Dressing

3 tbsp. lime juice

One diced or grated small piece of garlic

Three tablespoons extra virgin olive oil

1 tsp. raw honey

½ teaspoon whole grain

½ teaspoon of sea salt

Pepper

Directions

In a small frying pan, heat the ghee or coconut oil over medium to high heat. Add the onion and sauté for 4-5 minutes on medium heat, until golden. Attach the slimy chicken and garlic and swirl over medium-high heat for 2-3 minutes, breaking it apart.

Attach the turmeric, lime zest, lime juice, salt, and pepper, and cook for a further 3-4 minutes, stirring frequently. Set aside the cooked slush.

Bring a small saucepan of water to boil while the chicken cooks. Stir in the broccolini and cook for 2 minutes. Rinse under cold water, and cut into three to four pieces each.

Throw the pumpkin seeds from the chicken into the frying pan and toast for 2 minutes over medium heat, frequently stirring to prevent burning—season with a bit of salt. Deposit aside. Raw pumpkin seeds should also be used well.

In a salad bowl, place the chopped kale, and pour over the dressing. Toss the kale with the sauce, and rub it with your palms. It will soften the kale, kind of like what citrus juice does to carpaccio fish or beef—it' cooks' it a little bit.

The cooked rice, broccolini, fresh herbs, pumpkin seeds, and avocado slices are eventually tossed.

Nutrition

Calories: 1290 kcal

Protein: 131.39 g

Fat: 66.95 g

Carbohydrates: 40.87 g

13.   Buckwheat Noodles With Chicken Kale & Miso Dressing

Preparation time: 55 minutes

Cooking time: 20 minutes

Servings: 2

Ingredients

For Noodles

2-3 handfuls of kale leaves (removed from the stem and roughly cut)

Buckwheat noodles 150 g (5 oz.) (100% buckwheat, no wheat)

3-4 shiitake mushrooms, cut into slices

One teaspoon of coconut oil or ghee

One brown onion, finely diced

One medium free-range chicken breast, sliced or cubed

One long red chili, thinly chopped

Two large garlic cloves, finely diced

2-3 tablespoons of Tamari sauce (gluten-free soy sauce)

For miso dressing

1½ tbsp. fresh organic miso

1 tbsp. Tamari sauce

One tablespoon of extra virgin olive oil

One tablespoon lemon or lime juice

One teaspoon sesame oil

Directions

Bring a medium saucepan of boiling water. Attach the kale and cook until slightly wilted, for 1 minute. Remove and set aside, then bring the water back to the boil. Add the soba noodles and cook (usually about 5 minutes) according to packaging instructions. Set aside and rinse under cold water.

Meanwhile, in a little ghee or coconut oil (about a teaspoon), pan fry the shiitake mushrooms for 2-3 minutes, until lightly browned on either side. Sprinkle with salt from the sea, and set aside.

Heat more coconut oil or ghee in the same frying pan over medium to high heat. Stir in onion and chili for 2-3 minutes, and then add pieces of chicken. Cook over medium heat for 5 minutes, stirring a few times, and then add the garlic, tamari sauce, and some water splash. Cook for another 2-3 minutes, always stirring until chicken is cooked through.

Eventually, add the kale and soba noodles and warm up by stirring through the food. At the end of the cooking, mix the miso dressing and drizzle over the noodles, so you'll keep all those beneficial probiotics alive and active.

NutritionCalories: 256 kcalProtein: 10.82 gFat: 8.95 g Carbohydrates: 37.03 g

14. Asian King Prawn Stir-Fry With Buckwheat Noodles

Preparation time: 55 minutes

Cooking time: 20 minutes

Servings: 2

Ingredients

150g (5 ¼ oz.) raw royal shrimps in shelled skins

Two teaspoons of tamari (you can use soy sauce if you do not avoid gluten)

Two teaspoons extra virgin olive oil

75g (2 ¼ oz.) soba (buckwheat noodles)

One clove of garlic, finely chopped

One aerial view of finely chopped chili

One teaspoon of finely chopped fresh ginger

20g (¾ oz.) red onion, cut into slices

40g (1 ½ oz.) celery, trimmed and cut into slices

75g (2 ¼ oz.) chopped green beans

50g (1 ⅝ oz.) kale, coarsely chopped

100 ml (3.40 fl. oz.)of chicken stock

5g (3/16 oz.) lovage or celery leaves

Directions

Heat a frying pan over high heat, and then cook the prawns for 2–3 minutes in 1 teaspoon tamari and one teaspoon oil. Put the prawns on a plate. Wipe the pan out with paper from the oven, as you will be using it again.

Cook the noodles for 5–8 minutes in boiling water, or as indicated on the packet. Drain and put away. Meanwhile, over medium-high heat, fry the garlic, chili, ginger, red onion, celery, beans, and kale in the remaining oil for 2–3 minutes. Remove the stock and bring to the boil, then cook for one or two minutes until the vegetables are cooked but crunchy. Add the prawns, noodles, and leaves of lovage/celery to the pan, bring back to the boil, then remove the heat and serve.

Nutrition

Calories: 251 kcal

Protein: 22.97 g

Fat: 3.71 g

Carbohydrates: 34.14 g

15.   Choc Chip Granola

Preparation time: 55 minutes

Cooking time: 20 minutes

Servings: 2

Ingredients

200g (7 oz.) large oat flakes

Roughly 50 g (1 ⅝ oz.) pecan nuts chopped

Three tablespoons of light olive oil

20g (¾ oz.) butter

One tablespoon of dark brown sugar

2 tbsp. rice syrup

60 g (2 oz.) of good quality (70%) dark chocolate shavings

Directions

Oven preheats to 160°C (320°F) (140 ° C fan / Gas 3). Line a large baking tray with a sheet of silicone or parchment for baking.

In a large bowl, combine the oats and pecans. Heat the olive oil, butter, brown sugar, and rice malt syrup gently in a small non-stick pan until the butter has melted and the sugar and syrup dissolve. Do not let boil. Pour the syrup over the oats and stir thoroughly until fully covered with the oats.

Spread the granola over the baking tray and spread right into the corners. Leave the mixture clumps with spacing, instead of even laying. Bake for 20 minutes in the oven until golden brown is just tinged at the edges. Remove from the oven, and leave altogether to cool on the tray. When cold, split with your fingers any larger lumps on the tray and mix them in the chocolate chips. Put the granola in an airtight tub or jar, or pour it. The granola is to last for at least two weeks.

Nutrition

Calories: 914 kcal

Protein: 40.19 g

Fat: 63.05 g

Carbohydrates: 88.74 g

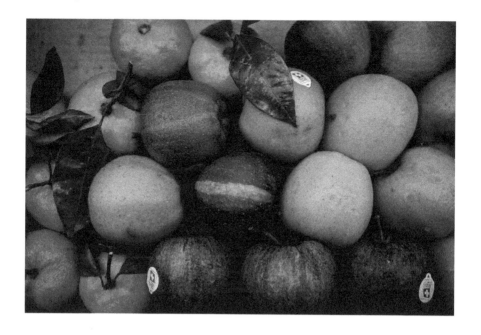

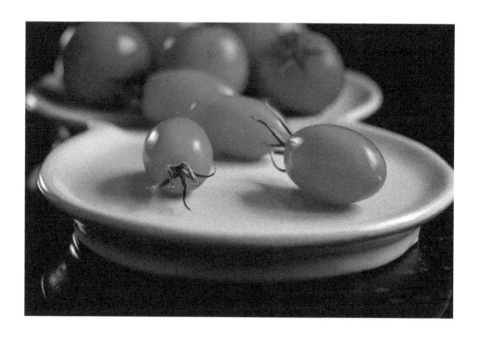

CHAPTER 7:

Dinner

16.   Sweet-Smelling Chicken Breast With Kale, Red Onion, And Salsa

Preparation Time: 15 Minutes

Cooking Time: 35 Minutes

Servings: 2

Ingredients

120g skinless, boneless chicken bosom

2 tsp. ground turmeric

Juice of ¼ lemon

tbsp. additional virgin olive oil

50g kale, slashed

20g red onion, cut

1tsp slashed new ginger

50g buckwheat

Directions:

To make the salsa, expel the tomato's eye and slash it finely, taking consideration to keep however much of the fluid as could reasonably be expected.

Blend in with the bean stew, tricks, parsley, and lemon juice. You could place everything in a blender, yet the final product is somewhat different.

Heat the broiler to 220°C/gas 7. Marinate the chicken bosom in 1 teaspoon of turmeric, lemon juice, and a little oil. Leave for 5–10 minutes.

Warmth an ovenproof griddle until hot, then include the marinated chicken and cook for a moment or so on each side, until pale brilliant, then exchange to the broiler (place on a preparing plate if your skillet isn't ovenproof) for 8–10 minutes or until cooked through.

Expel from the broiler, spread with foil, and leave to rest for 5 minutes before serving. In the meantime, cook the kale in a steamer for 5 minutes. Fry the red onions and the ginger in a little oil, until delicate however not shaded, including the cooked kale, and fry for one more moment.

Cook the buckwheat according to the parcel Directions with the rest of the teaspoon of turmeric. Serve nearby the chicken, vegetables, and salsa.

Nutrition:Calories 465Fat: 2 gCarbohydrates: 12 gProtein: 12 gFiber: 0 g

17.   Tuscan Bean Stew

Preparation Time: 15 minutes

Cooking Time: 40 minutes

Servings: 1

Ingredients

1tbsp. additional virgin olive oil

50g red onion, finely hacked

30g carrot, stripped and finely chopped

30g celery, cut and finely hacked

1garlic clove, finely hacked

½ 10,000 foot bean stew, finely slashed (discretionary)

1tsp herbs de Provence

200ml vegetable stock

1 x 400g tin hacked Italian tomatoes

1tsp tomato purée

200g tinned blended beans

50g kale, generally hacked

1tbsp. generally hacked parsley

40g buckwheat

Directions

Spot the oil in a medium pot over a low–medium warmth and delicately fry the onion, carrot, celery, garlic, chili (if utilizing) and herbs, until the onion is delicate yet not shaded.

Include the stock, tomatoes, and tomato purée and bring to the bubble. Include the beans and stew for 30 minutes.

Include the kale and cook for another 5–10 minutes, until delicate, then include the parsley. In the interim, cook the buckwheat according to the bundle Directions, deplete, and afterward present with the stew.

Nutrition:

Calories 289

Fat: 2 g

Carbohydrates: 10 g

Protein: 12 g

Fiber: 0 g

18.   Napa Cabbage Slaw

Preparation time: 10 minutes

Cooking time: 0 minutes

Servings: 4

Ingredients:

½ cup red bell pepper, cut into thin strips

One carrot, grated

4 cups Napa cabbage, shredded

Three green onions, chopped

One tablespoon olive oil

Two teaspoons ginger, grated

½ teaspoon red pepper flakes, crushed

Three tablespoons balsamic vinegar

One tablespoon coconut aminos

Three tablespoons low-fat peanut butter

Directions: In a salad bowl, mix bell pepper with carrot, cabbage, and onions and toss. Add oil, ginger, pepper flakes, vinegar, aminos, peanut butter, toss, divide into small cups and serve. Enjoy!

Nutrition: Calories 160 Fiber 3 Carbs 10 Protein 5

19.   Spiced Scrambled Eggs

Preparation Time: 2 minutes

Cooking Time: 10 minutes

Servings: 1

Ingredients:

One teaspoon extra virgin olive oil

1/8 cup (20g) red onion, finely chopped

1/2 Thai chili, finely chopped

Three medium eggs

1/4 cup (50ml) milk

One teaspoon ground turmeric

Two tablespoons (5g) parsley, finely chopped

Directions:

Heat the oil in a frying pan and fry the red onion and chili until soft but not browned.Whisk together the eggs, milk, turmeric, and parsley. Add to the hot pan and continue cooking over low to medium heat, continually moving the egg mixture around the pan to scramble it and stop it from sticking/burning. When you have achieved your desired consistency, serve.

Nutrition:Calories: 182 Cal Fat: 13 g Carbohydrates: 1 g Protein: 12 g

Fiber: 6 g

20.   Mushroom & Scrambled Tofu

Preparation Time: 10 min.

Cooking Time: 35 minutes

Servings: 4

Ingredients:

One teaspoonful of ground turmeric

⅙ of a cupful of red onion, thinly sliced

One cupful of mushrooms, thinly sliced

One teaspoonful of mild curry powder

4 ounces of extra-firm tofu

Two tablespoonful's of parsley, finely chopped

One teaspoonful of extra-virgin olive oil

⅓ of a cupful of kale, roughly chopped

½ chili, thinly sliced

Directions:

Cover the tofu with a paper towel and drain the excess moisture by placing a heavy item on it.

Pour the ground turmeric and teaspoonful of curry powder into an empty bowl and add some water. Mix until you get a puree. Then steam the chopped kale for 4 minutes.

Place a dry frypan over medium heat containing the teaspoonful of olive oil. Next, pour in the onion, cupful of mushroom, and thin slices of chili and fry for 4 minutes or until ingredients turn soft.

Crush the tofu into small bits and empty into the pan. Then spread in the pureed spice over the tofu surface and mix properly. Set stove heat to medium and cook for 4 minutes till the tofu just browns. Next, pour in the steamed kale and keep cooking for an extra minute. Lastly, empty in the chopped parsley and mix properly. Serve afterward.

Nutrition:

Energy (calories): 140 kcal

Protein: 12.15 g

Fat: 8.99 g

Carbohydrates: 6.1 g

CHAPTER 8:

Mains

21.   Filled Pita Pockets

Preparation Time: 20 minutes.

Cooking Time: 0 minutes

Servings: 1

Ingredients:

You need whole-grain pita bags.

For a filling with meat:

80g roasted turkey breast

25g rocket salad, finely chopped

20g cheese, grated

35g cucumbers, small diced

30g red onions, finely diced

15g walnuts, chopped

Dressing of 1 tablespoon balsamic vinegar and one tablespoon extra-virgin olive oil

For a vegan filling:

Three tablespoons hummus

35g cucumbers, small diced

30g red onions, finely diced

25g rocket salad, finely chopped

15g walnuts, chopped

Dressing of 1 tablespoon of extra virgin olive oil and some lemon juice

Direction:

In both variations, mix all the ingredients, fill the pita pockets with them, and marinate them with the dressing.

Nutrition:

Calories: 120

Fat: 1g.

Carbohydrate: 23g.

Protein: 21g.

22.   Lima Bean Dip With Celery And Crackers

Preparation Time: 10 minutes.

Cooking Time: 0 minutes

Servings: 2

Ingredients:

400g Lima beans or white beans from the tin

Three tablespoons of olive oil

Juice and zest of half an untreated lemon

Four spring onions, cut into fine rings

One garlic clove, pressed

1/4 Thai chili, chopped

Directions:

Drain the beans. Then mix all ingredients with a potato masher to a mass.

Serve with green celery sticks and crackers.

Nutrition:

Calories: 88

Fat: 0.7g.

Carbohydrates: 15.7g.Protein: 5.3g.

23.   Chili Con Carne

Preparation Time: 5 minutes.

Cooking Time: 30 minutes

Servings: 3

Ingredients:

One red onion, chopped

Three cloves of garlic, finely chopped

2 Tai chilies, finely chopped

One tablespoon of olive oil

One tablespoon turmeric

One tablespoon cumin

400g minced beef

150ml red wine

One red pepper, seeded and diced

Two cans of small tomatoes (400ml each)

One tablespoon of tomato paste

One tablespoon cocoa powder (without sugar)

150g canned kidney beans, drained

300ml beef broth

5g coriander green, chopped

5g parsley, chopped

160g buckwheat

Directions:

Sauté the onions, garlic, and chilies in olive oil in a high frying pan or a frying pan at medium heat. After three minutes, add cumin and turmeric and stir.

Then add the minced meat and fry until everything is brown. Add the red wine, bring to the boil and reduce by half.

Add the peppers, tomatoes, tomato paste, cocoa, kidney beans, and stock, stir and cook for an hour. Add a little water or broth if the chili is too dry.

Cook buckwheat according to the instructions on the packet and serve sprinkled with the chilies and fresh herbs.

Nutrition:

Calories 292.2 Fat: 11.0 g.

Carbohydrate: 20.0 g.

Protein: 26.0 g

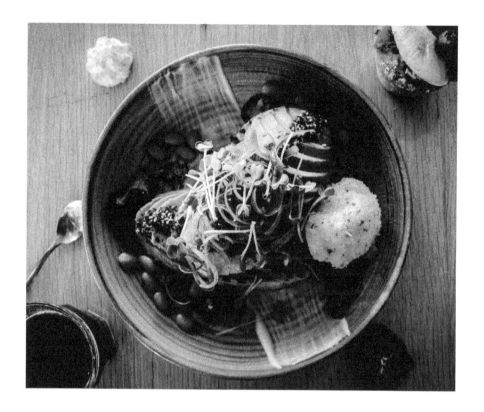

CHAPTER 9:

Meat

24.   Savory Chicken With Kale And Ricotta Salad

Preparation Time: 10 min.

Cooking Time: 40 minutes

Servings: 2

Ingredients:

 virgin olive oil, 1 tbsp.

One diced red onion

One finely chopped garlic cove

Juice and zest from ½ lemon

Diced chicken meat of your choosing, 300 g

A pinch of salt

A pinch of pepper

For salad

Pumpkin seeds, two tbsps.

Finely chopped kale, 2 cup

Ricotta cheese, ½ cup

Coriander leaves, chopped, ¼ cup

Parsley Leaves, chopped, ¼ cup

Salad dressing

Orange juice 3 tbsp.

One finely minced garlic clove

virgin olive oil, 3 tbsp.

Raw honey 1 tsp.

Wholegrain mustard ½ tsp.

A pinch of salt

A pinch of pepper

Directions:

Start by cooking chicken. Heat the oil over medium-high heat and add the onions. Let the onions sauté for up to five minutes. Once the onions turn a golden color, add the chicken and garlic if you'd like to finish quickly, stir-fry for up to three minutes at medium-high temperature, or lower the temperature and let it slowly simmer for up to fifteen minutes. The latter option will result in soft chicken, while the medium-heat stir fry will produce crunchy meat dices.

Next, add the lemon juice, pepper, zest, and turmeric during the last four cooking minutes. While your chicken is cooking, prepare the kale. While you can blanch the vegetable in boiling water for up to two minutes, I'd recommend microwaving with ½ cup of water for up to five minutes to preserve nutrients. Remember, kale is edible raw and cooking; it only serves to achieve the desired flavor and consistency. You can microwave the kale for as short as two minutes if all you need is for it to soften up, and the full five minutes if you prefer that fully-cooked taste.

During the last two minutes of chicken cooking, toss in the pumpkin seeds and stir fry. Remove from heat and set aside.

Mix both dishes into a bowl and add ricotta and the remaining fresh herbs. Enjoy!

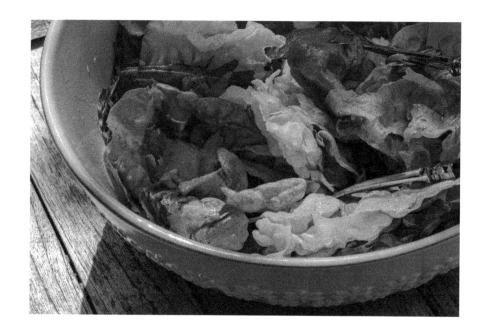

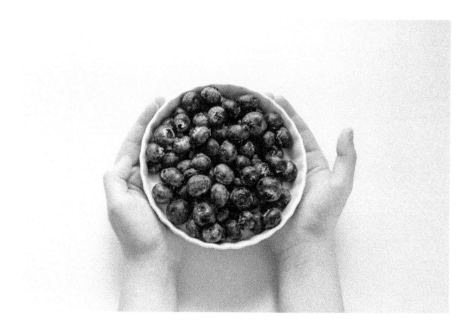

CHAPTER 10:

Sides

25. Vegan Wrap With Apples And Spicy Hummus

Preparation Time: 10 Minutes

Cooking Time: 0 Minutes

Servings: 2

INGREDIENTS:

One tortilla

6-7 tbsp. Spicy Hummus (mix it with a few tbsp. of salsa)

Only some leaves of fresh spinach or romaine lettuce

1 tsp. fresh lemon juice

1½ cups broccoli slaw

½ apple, sliced thin

4 tsp. dairy-free plain unsweetened yogurt

Salt and pepper

Directions:

Mix the yogurt and the lemon juice with the broccoli slaw. Add the salt and a dash of pepper for taste. Mix well and set aside.

Lay the tortilla flat.

Spread the spicy hummus over the tortilla.

Lay the lettuce down on the hummus.

On one half, pile the broccoli slaw on the lettuce.

Place the apple slices on the slaw.

Fold the tortilla sides up, starting with the end that has the apple and the slaw. Roll tightly.

Cut it in half and serve.

Nutrition:

Calories: 205 Fat: 2 g Protein: 12 g Carbs: 32 g Fiber: 9g

26.   Rice And Veggie Bowl

Preparation Time: 5 Minutes

Cooking Time: 15 Minutes

Servings: 6

Ingredients:

2 tbsp. coconut oil

1 tsp. ground cumin

1 tsp. ground turmeric

1 tsp. chili powder

One red bell pepper, chopped

1 tsp. tomato paste

One bunch of broccoli, cut into bite-sized florets with short stems

1 tsp. salt, to taste

One large red onion, sliced

Two garlic cloves, minced

One head of cauliflower, sliced into bite-sized florets

2 cups cooked rice

Newly ground black pepper to taste

Directions:

Heat the coconut grease over medium-high heat in a large pan

Wait until the oil is hot, stir in the turmeric, cumin, chili powder, salt, and tomato paste.

Cook the content for 1 minute. Stir repeatedly until the spices are fragrant.

Add the garlic and onion. Sauté for 3 minutes or until the onions are softened.

Add the broccoli, cauliflower, and bell pepper. Cover the pot. Cook for 3 to 4 minutes and stir occasionally.

Add the cooked rice. Stir so it will combine well with the vegetables—Cook for 2 to 3 minutes. Stir until the rice is warmed through.

Check the seasoning. And make adjustments to taste if desired.

Lower the heat and cook on low for 2 to 3 more minutes so the flavors will meld.

Serve with freshly ground black pepper.

Nutrition:

Calories: 260 Fat: 9 g Protein: 9 g Carbs: 36 g Fiber: 5g

27.   Roasted Asparagus

Preparation Time: 10 minutes.

Cooking Time: 10 minutes

Servings: 3

Ingredients:

One asparagus bunch, trimmed

3 tsp. avocado oil

A splash of lemon juice

Salt and ground black pepper to taste

1 tbsp. fresh oregano, chopped

Directions:

Spread the asparagus spears on a lined baking sheet, season with salt, and pepper, drizzle with oil and lemon juice, sprinkle with oregano and toss to coat well.

Put in an oven at 425°F, and bake for 10 minutes.

Divide onto plates and serve.

Nutrition: Calories 130 Fat 1 g Carbs 2 g Protein 3 g

28. Asparagus Frittata

Preparation Time: 10 minutes.

Cooking Time: 15 minutes

Servings: 4

Ingredients:

¼ cup onion, chopped

The drizzle of olive oil

1-pound asparagus spears, cut into 1-inch pieces

Salt and ground black pepper to taste

Four eggs whisked

1 cup cheddar cheese, grated

Directions:

Heat a pan with the oil over medium-high heat, add the onions, stir, and cook for 3 minutes. Add the asparagus, stir, and cook for 6 minutes. Add the eggs, stir, and cook for 3 minutes.

Add the salt and pepper, sprinkle with the cheese, put in an oven, and broil for 3 minutes.

Divide the frittata onto plates and serve.

Nutrition:

Calories 200 Fat 12 g Carbs 5 g Protein 14 g

CHAPTER 11:

Seafood

29.   Salmon With Asparagus Sauce

Preparation Time: 10 minutes

Cooking Time: 15 minutes

Servings: 2

Ingredients:

Two teaspoons olive oil

One tablespoon minced shallots

One garlic clove, minced

1/2 cup cooked chopped asparagus

1/2 teaspoon salt, divided

1/4 teaspoon white pepper, divided

Two teaspoons mayonnaise

1/4 teaspoon Dijon-style mustard

One salmon fillet,10 ounces

1/4 cup dry white wine

Two teaspoons grated Parmesan cheese

Directions:

In a 9-inch skillet, heat oil, add shallots and garlic, and sauté until shallots are translucent, careful not to burn the garlic.

Transfer shallot mixture to blender container. Add asparagus, 1/4 teaspoon salt, and 1/2 teaspoon pepper and process until smooth; set aside.

Preheat oven to 400°F. In a small bowl, combine mayonnaise and mustard; spread on fillet and sprinkle with remaining 1/4 teaspoon salt and 1/2 teaspoon pepper. Transfer salmon to 8 x 8 x 2-inch nonstick baking pan; add the wine and bake until fish flakes easily when tested with a fork, about 15 minutes (exact timing will depend upon the fillet's thickness).

Remove pan from oven and turn oven control to broil. Spread asparagus puree over fish and sprinkle with cheese. Broil just until heated through.

Nutrition:

Calories: 431 Cal

Fat: 28 g

Protein: 34 g

Sugar: 2.22 g

30. Batter And Fish

Preparation Time: 10 minutes

Cooking Time: 10 minutes

Servings: 2

Ingredients:

Three tablespoons all-purpose flour

1/4 teaspoon double-acting baking powder

1/2s teaspoon salt

Three tablespoons water

10 ounces scrod fillets, cut into 1-inch pieces

One tablespoon plus one teaspoon vegetable oil

Sweet 'n' Sour Medley

1/22 cup diagonally sliced carrot (thin slices)

1/4 cup water

1/2 cup canned pineapple chunks (no sugar added), drain and reserve juice

1/4 cup each diced red and green bell peppers

Two teaspoons each firmly packed

brown sugar and teriyaki sauce

One teaspoon each cornstarch and rice wine vinegar

1/2 teaspoon salt

Directions:

To Prepare Sweet 'n' Sour Medley: In 1-quart saucepan, combine carrot and water; bring to a boil. Reduce heat, cover, and let simmer until carrot slices are tender, about 3 minutes; stir in pineapple chunks and red and green peppers and cook until mixture is heated. In measuring cup or small bowl, combine reserved pineapple juice with remaining ingredients for sweet 'n' sour medley, stirring to dissolve cornstarch; pour over carrot mixture and cook, and continue stirring mixture thickens and is thoroughly heated. Set aside.

To Prepare Fish: In a small bowl, using a fork, combine dry ingredients, add water and stir until batter is smooth. Add fish pieces to the batter and turn until thoroughly coated.

In 10-inch nonstick skillet, heat oil over medium-high heat; add fish and cook until golden brown on the bottom, 3 to 4 minutes. Carefully turn pieces over and cook until another side is browned; remove to a serving platter and top with warm sweet 'n' sour medley.

Nutrition:

Calories: 323 Cal Fat: 11 g

Protein: 27 g

Sugar: 28.85 g

CHAPTER 12:

Poultry

31.   Chicken In Sweet And Sour Sauce With Corn Salad

Preparation time: 10 minutes

Cooking time: 45 minutes

Servings: 4

Ingredients

2 cups plus two tablespoons of unflavored low-fat yogurt

2 cups of frozen mango chunks

Three tablespoons of honey

¼ cup plus one tablespoon apple cider vinegar

¼ cup sultana

Two tablespoons of olive oil, plus an amount to be brushed

¼ teaspoon of cayenne pepper

Five dried tomatoes (not in oil)

Two small cloves of garlic, finely chopped

Four cobs, peeled

Eight peeled and boned chicken legs, peeled (about 700g)

Halls

6 cups of mixed salad

Two medium carrots, finely sliced

Directions:

For the smoothie: in a blender, mix 2 cups of yogurt, 2 cups of ice, 1 cup of mango, and all the honey until the mixture becomes completely smooth. Divide into four glasses and refrigerate until ready to use. Rinse the blender.

Preheat the grill to medium-high heat. Mix the remaining cup of mango, ¼ cup water, ¼ cup vinegar, sultanas, olive oil, cayenne pepper, tomatoes, and garlic in a microwave bowl. Cover with a transparent film and cook in the microwave until the tomatoes become soft, for about 3 minutes. Leave to cool slightly and pass in a blender. Transfer to a small bowl. Leave two tablespoons aside to garnish, turn the chicken into the remaining mixture.

Place the corn on the grill, cover, and bake, turning it over if necessary, until it is burnt, about 10 minutes. Remove and keep warm.

Brush the grill over medium heat and brush the grills with a little oil. Turn the chicken legs into half the remaining sauce and ½ teaspoon of salt. Place on the grill and cook until the cooking marks appear and the internal temperature reaches 75°C on an instantaneous thermometer, 8 to 10 minutes per side. Bart and sprinkle a few times with the remaining sauce while cooking.

While the chicken is cooking, beat the remaining two tablespoons of yogurt, the two tablespoons of sauce set aside, the remaining spoonful of vinegar, one tablespoon of water, and ¼ teaspoon of salt in a large bowl. Mix the mixed salad with the carrots. Divide chicken, corn, and salad into four serving dishes. Garnish the salad with the dressing set aside. Serve each plate with a mango smoothie.

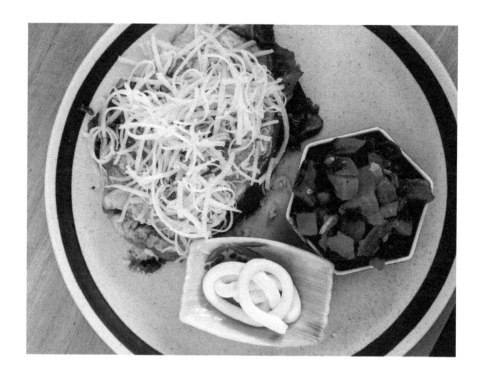

CHAPTER 13:

Vegetable

32. May Beet Salad With Cucumber

Preparation Time: 8 min.

Cooking Time: 20 minutes

Servings: 2

Ingredients:

3 May turnips

One cucumber

One onion

2 stems parsley

150 g Greek yogurt

1 tbsp. fruit crush vinegar

1 tsp. nectar

1 tsp. mustard

Sea-salt

Cayenne pepper

Pepper

Directions:

Clean, strip, and cut the turnips. Clean and wash the cucumber and slicer. Clean, wash, and cut the spring onions into rings. Put everything during a serving of mixed greens bowl and blend.

Wash parsley, shake dry, and slash finely. Combine dressing with yogurt, fruit crush vinegar, nectar, mustard, and 2–3 tbsp. Water. Season with salt and cayenne pepper.

Mix the plate of mixed greens dressing with the mayonnaise and cucumber and let it steep for around 10 minutes. At that point, crush it with pepper and serve.

33. Ricotta Pancakes With Apricots

Preparation Time: 10 min.

Cooking Time: 20 minutes

Servings: 2

Ingredients:

80 g ricotta

One egg

3 tbsp. juice

1 tsp. nectar

40 g buckwheat flour

½ tsp. preparing powder

1 tsp. coconut oil

Two apricots

3 tbsp. yogurt (3.5% fat)

One stem mint

Directions:

Mix the ricotta with the egg, lemon squeeze, and nectar until smooth. Include buckwheat flour and preparing powder and blend into a gooey mixture. Warmth coconut oil during a container and include a massive tablespoon of hitter to the dish, steel oneself against one moment over medium warmth, divert, and keep heating from the opposite side. Do likewise for around five flapjacks.

Within the interim, wash, split, and cut apricots. Blend the yogurt until velvety. Wash mint, shake dry and pluck leaves. Stack the flapjacks on a plate, including the yogurt and apricot wedges, and serve improved with mint.

34. Buddha Bowl With Green Asparagus And Soba Noodles

Preparation Time: 10 min.

Cooking Time: 25 minutes

Servings: 4

Ingredients:

125 g soba noodle (buckwheat noodles)

Salt

Two bunches of child spinach (40 g)

½ pack youthful radishes

100 g sugar snap

200 g green asparagus

1 tbsp. oil

1 tbsp. tahini (15 g)

2 tbsp. juice

Pepper

One nectarine

75 g feta

2 tsp. dark sesame (10 g)

Directions:

Cook soba noodles in bubbling salted water in 4–5 minutes, channel, extinguish with cold water, and drain. Clean and wash infant spinach, radishes, and sugar snap peas. Cut the sugar snap unit lengthways.

Clean, wash and cut green asparagus.

Warmth 1 tablespoon of oil during a container and fry the asparagus in it over medium heat for five minutes.

Meanwhile, mix the tahini with juice until smooth and blend in enough water until the consistency is adequate fluid. Season the sauce with salt and pepper.

Wash, divide, expel the center and cut the nectarine into wedges.

Disintegrate the feta. Spread the soba noodles, all vegetables, nectarine cuts on two dishes, and serve beat with tahini sauce, feta, and dark sesame.

CHAPTER 14:

Soup, Curries and Stews

35. Parsley Soup

Preparation Time: 10 min.

Cooking Time: 20 minutes

Servings: 4

Ingredients:

One bunch of parsley

One small zucchini

½ leek, white portion only

½ teaspoon kosher salt

Three tablespoons olive oil

¼ cup red wine

½ teaspoon freshly ground black pepper

½ cup chicken broth

Directions:

Cut the leek into small pieces. Rinse and pat dry. Set aside.

Cut the zucchini into slices. Set aside.

Chop the parsley and set aside.

Heat olive oil in a large saucepan. Add parsley and leek, sauté for 2-3 minutes on medium flame.

Add zucchini and salt. Stir-fry for about 4-5 minutes.

Add chicken broth and red wine. Stir well.

Cover the saucepan with a lid. Simmer the mixture on medium to low flame for about 6-8 minutes.

Puree the mixture in a blender.

Season soup with as much black pepper as desired.

Transfer soup to serving dish.

Garnish with the desired ingredient.

Serve hot

Enjoy.

Nutrition:

Calories – 671

Fat – 54 g

Carbs – 0.5 g Protein – 39 g

36.   Kale And Walnut Soup

Preparation Time: 5 min.

Cooking Time: 20 minutes

Servings: 4

Ingredients:

2 lbs. kale leaves

One small red onion, sliced

4-5 medium garlic cloves, minced

7-8 walnuts, chopped

½ cup chicken broth

One green chili, sliced

½ teaspoon kosher salt

0.2 lb. goat cheese

3-4 tablespoons olive oil

Directions:

Chop the kale leaves. Set aside.

Cut the onions into slices. Set aside.

Chop the walnuts, set aside.

Heat olive oil In a large saucepan. Add onion and sauté until softened.

Add kale leaves, salt, and garlic. Stir-fry kale leaves for about 3-4 minutes.

Add chicken broth and stir well—season with black pepper. Let to simmer for about 8-10 minutes on low flame.

Add goat cheese and mix well. Add walnuts and mix well.

Puree the mixture in a blender.

Transfer soup to serving dish.

Garnish with the desired ingredient.

Serve hot and enjoy.

Nutrition:

Calories – 673

Fat – 645 g

Carbs – 212 g

Protein – 241 g

37.   French Onion Soup

Preparation time: 10 minutes

Cooking time: 65 minutes

Servings: 4

Ingredients

1 tbsp. of olive oil

2 slices of wholemeal bread

750 g red onions (thinly sliced)

2 tsp. of flour

900 ml beef stock

12 g butter

50 g cheddar cheese (shredded)

Directions

Place a saucepan over high heat and add butter to melt and heat up.

Add onions to the pan and reduce the heat to low. Cook for 25 minutes while stirring continuously.

Add flour and stir thoroughly.

Add beef stock and stir. Bring to a boil.

Reduce heat and allow the soup to simmer for 30 minutes.

Remove from heat.

Sprinkle cheese on the bread slices and grill them until the cheese melts.

Serve soup with cheesy bread slices on top.

Nutrition:

Energy (calories): 2736 kcal

Protein: 134.63 g

Fat: 231.56 g

Carbohydrates: 29.1 g

CHAPTER 15:

Snacks & Desserts

38.   Mascarpone Cheesecake With Almond Crust

Preparation time: 20 minutes

Cooking time: 25 minutes

Servings: 4

Ingredients:

Crust:

1/2 cup slivered almonds

Eight teaspoons or 2/3 cups graham cracker crumbs

Two tablespoons sugar

One tablespoon salted butter melted

Filling:

1 (8-ounce) package cream cheese, room temperature

1 (8-ounce) container mascarpone cheese, room temperature

3/4 cups sugar

One teaspoon fresh lemon juice (or imitation lemon-juice)

One teaspoon vanilla infusion

Two large eggs, room temperature

Directions:

For the crust:

Preheat oven to 350°F. Take per 9-inch diameter around the pan. Finely grind the almonds, cracker crumbs, sugar in a food processor. Bring the butter and process until moist crumbs form.

Press the almond mixture on the prepared pan's base (maybe not on the pan's surfaces). Bake the crust until it is put and starts to brown, about 1-2 minutes. Cool. Decrease the oven temperature to 325°F.

For your filling:

With an electric mixer, beat the cream cheese, mascarpone cheese, and sugar in a large bowl until smooth, occasionally scraping down the sides of the jar using a rubber spatula. Beat in the lemon juice and vanilla. Add the eggs, one at a time, beating until combined after each addition.

Pour the cheese mixture on the crust from the pan. Put the pan into a big skillet or Pyrex dish; pour enough hot water into the roasting pan to come halfway up the sides of one's skillet. Bake until the middle of this racket goes slightly when the pan is gently shaken, about 1 hour (the dessert will get business if it's cold). Transfer the cake to a stand; trendy for 1 hour. Refrigerate until the cheesecake is out, at least eight hours.

Topping squeezed just a small thick cream in the microwave using a damaged chocolate brown—afterward, get a plastic bag and cut out a hole at the corner—then pour the melted chocolate to the baggie and use this to decorate the cake!

Nutrition:

Kcal 534

Net carbs 18 g

Fat 22 g

Fiber 17 g

Protein 32 g

39.   Marshmallow Popcorn Balls

Preparation time: 5 minutes

Cooking time: 10 minutes

Servings: 16

Ingredients:

Two bags of microwave popcorn

1 12.6 ounces tote M&M's

3 cups honey roasted peanuts

One package of 16-ounce massive marshmallows

1 cup butter, cubed

Directions:

In a bowl, blend the popcorn, peanuts, and M&M's.

In a big pot, combine marshmallows and butter. Cook medium-low warmth. Insert popcorn mix, blend nicely Spray muffin tins with nonstop cooking spray. When cool enough to handle, spray hands together with non-stick cooking spray and then shape into chunks and put into the muffin tin to carry contour. Add Popsicle stick into each chunk and then let cool. Wrap each person in vinyl when chilled.

Nutrition:

Kcal 300 Net carbs 24 g

Fat 23 g Fiber 34 g Protein 30 g

40. Homemade Ice-Cream Drumsticks

Preparation time: 25 minutes

Cooking time: 0 minutes

Servings: 2

Ingredients:

Vanilla ice cream

Two hazelnut chunks

A magical shell of chocolate

Sugar levels

Nuts

Parchment newspaper

Directions:

Soften the ice cream and mix the topping (two sliced hazel nutballs).

Fill underside of sugar with magic and nutshells and top with ice-cream.

Wrap parchment paper round cone and then fill cone over about 1.5 inches across the cone's cap (the newspaper can help carry its shape), shirt with magical nuts and shells.

Freeze for about 20 minutes before ice-cream is business.

Nutrition: Kcal 546Net carbs 25 g Fat 20 g Fiber 21 g Protein 18 g

41. Ultimate Chocolate Chip Cookie Fudge Brownie Bar

Preparation time: 25 minutes

Cooking time: 40 minutes

Servings: 2

Ingredients:

1 cup (2 sticks) butter, softened

1 cup granulated sugar

3/4 cup light brown sugar

Two big eggs

One tablespoon pure vanilla extract

2 1/2 cups all-purpose flour

One teaspoon baking soda

One teaspoon lemon

2 cups (12 ounces) milk chocolate chips

Inch per kg double stuffed Oreos

Inch family-size (9×1-3) brownie mixture

1/4 cup hot fudge topping

Directions:

Preheat oven to 350°F.

Mix the butter and sugars in a large bowl, using an electric mixer at medium speed for 35 minutes.

Add the vanilla and eggs and mix well to combine thoroughly. In another bowl, whisk together the flour, baking soda, salt, and slowly incorporate it into the mixer until the bread is simply connected.

Stir in chocolate chips.

Spread the cookie dough at the bottom of a 9×1-3 baking dish wrapped with wax paper and then coated with cooking spray, shirt with a coating of Oreos.

Mix brownie mix, adding an optional 1/4 cup of hot fudge directly into the mixture.

Twist the brownie batter within the cookie-dough and Oreos.

Cover with foil and bake at 350°F for half an hour.

Remove foil and continue baking for another 15-25 minutes. Let cool before cutting on brownies might nevertheless be gooey at the midst while warm, but will also place up perfectly once chilled.

Nutrition:

Kcal 490 Net carbs 29 g Fat 27 g Fiber 16 g

Protein 32 g

42.   Cauliflower Nachos

Preparation Time: 5 min.

Cooking Time: 25 minutes

Servings: 4

Ingredients:

Two tablespoons extra virgin olive oil

½ teaspoon onion powder

½ teaspoon turmeric

½ teaspoon ground cumin

One large head cauliflower

¾ cup shredded cheddar cheese

½ cup tomato, diced

¼ cup red bell pepper, diced

¼ cup red onion, diced

½ Bird's Eye chili pepper, finely diced

¼ cup parsley, finely diced

Pinch of salt

Directions:

Preheat oven to 400° F.

Mix the onion powder, cumin, turmeric, and olive oil.

Core cauliflower and slice into ½"-thick rounds.

Coat the cauliflower with the olive oil mixture and bake for 15-20 minutes.

Top with shredded cheese and bake for an additional 3-5 minutes, until cheese is melted.

In a bowl, combine tomatoes, bell pepper, onion, chili, and parsley with a salt pinch.

Top cooked cauliflower with salsa and serve.

Nutrition:

140Calories Total Fat 7g

Carbohydrate 19g Protein1g

43. Cardamom Granola Bars

Preparation Time: 10 min.

Cooking Time: 30 min. +30 min. Cooling

Servings: 18 bars

Ingredients:

2 cups rolled oats

½ cup raisins

½ cup walnuts, chopped and toasted

1½ teaspoons ground cardamom

Six tablespoons cocoa butter

1/3 cup packed brown sugar

Three tablespoons honey Coconut oil, for greasing pan

Directions:

Preheat oven to 350° F.

Line a 9-inch square pan with foil, extending the foil over the sides. Grease the foil with coconut oil.

Mix the oats, raisins, walnuts, and cardamom in a large bowl.

Heat the cocoa butter, brown sugar, and honey in a saucepan until the butter melts and begins to bubble. Pour this mixture over the dry ingredients and mix until well coated. Transfer to the prepared pan and press evenly with a spatula. Bake for 30 minutes or until the top is golden brown. Allow cooling for 30 minutes. Using the foil, lift the granola out of the pan and place it on the cutting board.

Cut into 18 bars.

Nutrition:

Energy (calories): 1194 kcal

Protein: 39.1 g Fat: 53.1 g

Carbohydrates: 220.79 g

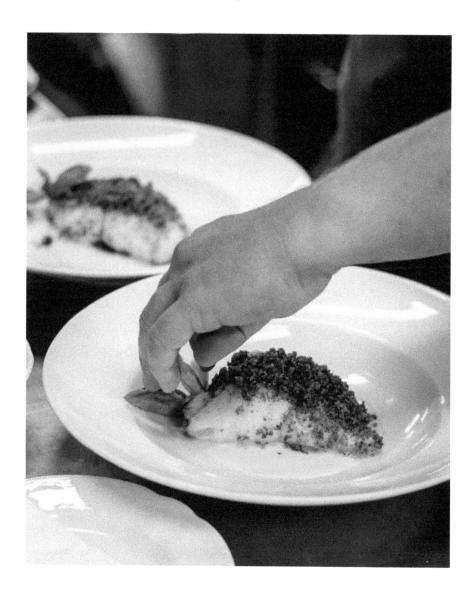

CHAPTER 16:

Desserts

44.   Chocolate Balls

Preparation Time: 5 Minutes

Cooking time: 25 Minutes Servings: 2

Ingredients

50g (2oz) peanut butter (or almond butter)

25g (1oz) cocoa powder

25g (1oz) desiccated (shredded) coconut

1 tablespoon honey

1 tablespoon cocoa powder for coating

Directions: Place the ingredients into a bowl and mix. Using a teaspoon, scoop out a little of the mixture and shape it into a ball. Roll the ball in a little cocoa powder and set aside. Repeat for the remaining mixture. It can be eaten straight away or stored in the fridge.

Nutrition:Energy   (calories):   435   kcalProtein: 18.04   gFat: 18.51gCarbohydrates: 57.19 g

45.   Warm Berries & Cream

Preparation Time: 5 Minutes

Cooking time: 45 Minutes

Servings: 2

Ingredients

250g (9oz) blueberries

250g (9oz) strawberries

100g (3½ oz.) redcurrants

100g (3½ oz.) blackberries

Four tablespoons fresh whipped cream

One tablespoon honey

Zest and juice of 1 orange

Directions:

Place all of the berries into a pan along with the honey and orange juice. Gently heat the berries for around 5 minutes until warmed through.

Serve the berries into bowls and add a dollop of whipped cream on top. Alternatively, you could top them off with fromage frais or yogurt.

Nutrition:

Energy (calories): 485 kcal

Protein: 5.08 g Fat: 4.61 g Carbohydrates: 115.3 g

46.   Chocolate Fondue

Preparation Time: 5 Minutes

Cooking time: 35 Minutes

Servings: 2

Ingredients

125g (4oz) dark chocolate (min 85% cocoa)

300g (11oz) strawberries

200g (7oz) cherries

Two apples, peeled, cored, and sliced

100mls (3½ fl. oz.) double cream (heavy cream)

Directions:

Place the chocolate and cream into a fondue pot or saucepan and warm it until smooth and creamy. Serve in the fondue pot or transfer it to a serving bowl. Scatter the fruit on a serving dish, ready to be dipped into the chocolate.

Nutrition: Cholesterol 11mg Calories510 Total Fat 42.3g

Saturated Fat 12.5g Sodium 39mg

Total Carbohydrate 29.5g

Dietary Fiber 0.6g

Sugars 25.6g Protein3.8g

47.   Walnut & Date Loaf

Preparation Time: 5 Minutes

Cooking time: 45 Minutes

Servings: 2

Ingredients

250g (9oz) self-rising flour

125g (4oz) Medjool dates, chopped

50g (2oz) walnuts, chopped

250mls (8fl oz.) milk

Three eggs

One medium banana, mashed

One teaspoon baking soda

Directions:

Sieve the baking soda and flour into a bowl. Add in the banana, eggs, milk, and dates and combine all the ingredients thoroughly. Transfer the mixture to a lined loaf tin and smooth it out. Scatter the walnuts on top. Bake the loaf in the oven at 180C/360F for 45 minutes. Transfer it to a wire rack to cool before serving.

Nutrition:Energy (calories): 1793 kcal Protein: 44.86 g Fat: 45.25 g Carbohydrates: 314.08 g

48.   Chocolate Brownies

Preparation Time: 5 Minutes

Cooking time: 35 Minutes

Servings: 2

Ingredients

200g (7oz) dark chocolate (min 85% cocoa)

200g (70z) medjool dates, stone removed

100g (3½oz) walnuts, chopped

3 eggs

25mls (1fl oz.) melted coconut oil

2 teaspoons vanilla essence

½ teaspoon baking soda

Directions:

Place the dates, chocolate, eggs, coconut oil, baking soda, and vanilla essence into a food processor and mix until smooth. Stir the walnuts into the mixture. Pour the mixture into a shallow baking tray.

Transfer to the oven and bake at 180C/350F for 25-30 minutes. Allow it to cool. Cut into pieces and serve. Nutrition:70Calories Total Fat 3g Saturated Fat 1gTrans Fat 0g Cholesterol 0mg Protein2g

49.   Mango Banana Drink With Fruit Juice And Yogurt

Preparation time: 10 minutes

Cooking time: 0 minutes

Servings: 1

Ingredients:

Five juice oranges

One little ready mango

One ready banana

150 g yogurt (3.5% fat)

Directions:

Halve and press oranges.

Peel the mango. Cut the mash into cuts from the stone and usually dice.

Peel the banana and break it into pieces. Puree with squeezed orange, mango pieces, and yogurt during a blender (or with a hand blender). Fill in 2 glasses (300 ml each).

Nutrition:

Calories: 171 kcal

Protein: 21.69 g

Fat: 6.65

Carbohydrates: 5.4 g

50.   Yogurt With Berries, Chocolate, And Brazil Nuts

Preparation time: 10 minutes

Cooking time: 0 minutes

Servings: 1

Ingredients:

400 g yogurt (3.5% fat)

150 g strawberries

100 g blueberries

40 g dull chocolate (in any event 70% cocoa)

50 g Brazil nut piece

2 tsp. flaxseed oil

Directions:

Stir yogurt until smooth and partition into two dishes. Clean, wash and slash strawberries. Wash and touch the blueberries.

Roughly slash dim chocolate and Brazil nuts. Put the berries on the yogurt. Sprinkle with chocolate and nuts, and shower with the flaxseed oil.

Nutrition:

Calories: 975 kcal

Protein: 56.85 g Fat: 51.41 g Carbohydrates: 79.93 g

51.   Strawberry Spinach Smoothie

Preparation time: 10 minutes

Cooking time: 0 minutes

Servings: 1

Ingredients:

1 cup entire solidified strawberries

3 cups pressed spinach

¼ cup solidified pineapple lumps

One medium ready banana, dig lumps and solidified

1 cup unsweetened milk

One tablespoon chia seeds

Directions:

Place all the fixings during a powerful blender.

Blend until smooth.

Enjoy!

Nutrition:

Calories 266, Fat 8g,

Carbohydrates 48g,

Protein 9g

Conclusions

Most diets have been proven to be just a temporary fix. If you want to keep weight off for a good while maintaining muscle mass and ensuring that your body stays healthy, then you need to be following a diet that activates your sirtuin genes: in other words, the Sirtfood Diet.

Sirtuins play an essential role in burning body fat and also help to increase the metabolic rate. But sirtuin genes aren't just responsible for weight loss and muscle gain—they also help prevent illnesses such as heart disease, diabetes, bone problems, Alzheimer's, and even cancer. To activate these genes, you must eat foods that are high in the plant-based proteins polyphenols.

It is essential to eat a diet that combines whole, healthy, nutritious ingredients with various sirtfoods. These ingredients will all work together to increase the bioavailability of the sirtfoods even further. And there's no need to count calories: just focus on sensible portions and consume a diverse range of foods—including as many sirtfoods as you can and eating until you feel full.

You should also ensure you have a green sirtfood-rich juice every day to get all of those sirtuins- activating ingredients into your body. Also, feel free to indulge in tea, coffee, and the occasional glass of red wine. And most importantly, be adventurous. Now is the time to start leading a happy, healthy, and fat-free life without having to deprive you of delicious and satisfying food.